MENOPAUSE MASTERY

Holistic Therapies for a Smooth Transition

Empower Women With Effective And Natural Therapies To Manage The Symptoms Of Menopause And Maintain Overall Well-Being

DR. BRIDGET PROMISE

Table of Contents

CHAPTER ONE

Introduction

Menopause is a regular organic procedure that ends a woman's reproductive years. Menopause, which often occurs in the late 40s or early 50s, is marked by the end of menstruation as well as a sequence of hormonal changes that cause numerous physical and emotional upheavals.

While menopause is a common experience for women, each person's path through it is unique. In this examination, we will look at the complexities of menopause, including the physiological elements, typical symptoms, and problems that women may experience throughout this transition. We will also examine holistic methods of menopausal management, highlighting the need to treat physical, mental, and lifestyle components to provide a well-rounded and empowered experience.

Understanding Menopause

Menopause is a normal period of a woman's life that marks the end of her reproductive years. It is formally diagnosed after 12 months without a menstrual cycle. Perimenopause is the period before menopause when hormonal swings become more apparent. Estrogen and progesterone, two essential hormones in the menstrual cycle, alter dramatically throughout this period.

During menopause, estrogen levels fall, which are important for regulating the menstrual cycle and preserving bone density. Progesterone, the hormone responsible for preparing the uterus for pregnancy, also drops. The combined effects of these hormone fluctuations may cause a variety of physical and emotional changes.

Hormonal Shift: What Happens During Menopause

Menopause is mostly caused by the natural aging process, in which the ovaries progressively lower the synthesis of estrogen and progesterone.

The hormonal imbalance that follows causes many physiological changes that signal the menopausal transition.

One noticeable impact is the irregularity of menstrual periods during perimenopause. Women may have shorter or longer cycles, skipped periods, or more or less bleeding. Another typical symptom is hot flashes, which are defined as abrupt and powerful waves of heat. These may be accompanied by nocturnal sweats, which impair sleep patterns.

Changes in hormone levels influence bone health. Estrogen is essential for maintaining bone density, and its loss after menopause may contribute to the development of osteoporosis. Maintaining bone health with a well-balanced diet and frequent exercise is critical throughout this stage.

Hormonal variations may have an impact on both vaginal and urinary health. Reduced estrogen levels may cause vaginal dryness and weakening of the vaginal walls, resulting in pain and an increased risk of urinary tract infections. Addressing these problems is critical to sustaining overall health during and after menopause.

Common Symptoms And Challenges.

Menopause causes several symptoms, which vary in strength and length for each woman. Aside from the physiological changes stated above, menopausal symptoms might include emotional and psychological components.

Mood swings, anger, and anxiety are prevalent throughout menopause. Hormonal variations may alter neurotransmitters in the brain, affecting mood regulation. Furthermore, physical symptoms such as hot flashes and night sweats may cause sleep difficulties, resulting in weariness and heightened emotional sensitivity.

Menopause might also provide challenges in keeping a healthy weight. A drop in estrogen levels might change the distribution of body fat, increasing the risk of weight gain, especially around the belly. This shift in body composition, along with a natural slowdown of metabolism with age, necessitates a careful approach to nutrition and exercise to successfully control weight.

CHAPTER TWO

Holistic Approaches To Menopause

Given the varied nature of menopause, addressing its issues requires a comprehensive strategy that includes physical, mental, and behavioral factors.

1. Nutrition and Exercise: During menopause, a balanced and nutritious diet is essential for maintaining overall health. Maintaining bone density requires an adequate diet of calcium and vitamin D. Regular exercise, especially weight-bearing exercises, helps to maintain bone

health and manage weight. Additionally, physical exercise helps to enhance mood and sleep.

2. Mind-Body Practices: Yoga, meditation, and deep breathing techniques may help manage stress and promote emotional well-being. These approaches not only assist with mood swings and anxiety, but they also improve sleep quality.

3. Hormone Replacement Therapy (HRT): Some women may benefit from hormone replacement therapy to relieve severe menopausal symptoms. HRT includes giving the body estrogen

or a mixture of estrogen and progesterone. However, it is important to examine the possible dangers and advantages with a healthcare physician, since HRT may not be appropriate for everyone.

4. Herbal Remedies: Some women utilize herbal supplements to relieve menopausal symptoms. Black cohosh, red clover, and evening primrose oil are among the plants widely used to treat symptoms. However, it is important to speak with a healthcare expert before adopting herbal therapies into one's daily

regimen to ensure safety and effectiveness.

5. therapy and Support Groups: Menopause's emotional issues may be successfully handled by therapy or involvement in support groups. Sharing your experiences with others who are going through similar changes might help you feel more connected and understood.

Menopause is a transforming journey that ends one stage of a woman's life and begins another. Understanding the physiological changes, typical symptoms, and obstacles of menopause is critical for making the transition with grace and fortitude. Holistic techniques that include diet, exercise, mind-body practices, and, when required, medical treatments may all help to create a pleasant and empowered menopause experience.

Women may enter this new chapter with confidence and well-being if they embrace the changes and manage the physical and mental components of menopause ahead of time.

Nutritional Strategies For Hormone Balance

Achieving hormonal balance is critical for general health, especially during major life changes like menopause. Nutritional methods are essential for maintaining hormonal balance. A well-balanced diet may help control hormone swings and lessen their effects.

For starters, adopting a range of nutrient-dense meals is critical. Foods high in omega-3 fatty acids, such as fatty fish, flaxseeds, and walnuts, aid in hormone balance. Omega-3 fatty acids help to reduce inflammation and boost brain function, both of which may improve hormonal balance.

Furthermore, adding an adequate number of high-fiber foods to the diet is critical. Fiber helps to keep blood sugar constant and may help control insulin resistance, which is typically associated with hormonal abnormalities. Fiber-rich foods include whole grains, legumes, fruits, and vegetables.

Eating a variety of colored fruits and vegetables is also good. These foods are high in antioxidants, vitamins, and minerals, all of which help the body operate properly, including hormone control. Cruciferous vegetables, like broccoli and kale, contain chemicals that aid in estrogen metabolism.

Furthermore, eating lean proteins like chicken, fish, tofu, and beans promotes muscle health and satiety. Adequate protein consumption is essential for hormone synthesis and may aid with weight management, which is often linked to hormonal balance.

Herbal Remedy and Supplement:

Herbal medicines and supplements are becoming more well-recognized for their ability to naturally promote hormonal balance. While it is important to contact a healthcare expert before starting any new supplements, some choices have shown potential in treating hormonal issues.

Black cohosh is a popular plant for treating menopausal symptoms. According to research, black cohosh may help decrease hot flashes and nocturnal sweats, giving women comfort from hormonal changes.

Another herbal medicine that has grown in favor is maca root, which is native to the Andes Mountains and has been shown to improve hormonal health. Maca is thought to affect the endocrine system and assist in regulating hormones, especially in women going through menopause.

Vitex, often known as chasteberry, is a plant that has long been used to help women's reproductive health. It may help regulate menstrual cycles and relieve symptoms linked with hormonal imbalances, making it a useful ally at many periods of life.

In addition to herbal therapies, several vitamins may aid with hormonal balance. Omega-3 fatty acid supplements, for example, might be a handy approach to improve consumption for those who don't eat fish or flaxseeds daily. Vitamin D is another important vitamin since it regulates hormones and promotes general health.

Mind-Body Techniques For Emotional Wellbeing:

Emotional well-being is inextricably related to hormonal balance, particularly during times of hormonal shifts such as menopause. Mind-body techniques are powerful methods for stress reduction, relaxation, and emotional balance.

Mindfulness meditation, which involves concentrating on the present moment without judgment, has been demonstrated to reduce stress and improve emotional well-being. Incorporating mindfulness into everyday activities may help women deal with the emotional issues that come with hormonal changes.

Yoga, which combines physical postures, breathing exercises, and meditation, is another beneficial mind-body activity. Regular yoga practice has been linked to decreased stress and enhanced mood, which helps to maintain emotional stability amid hormonal transitions.

Cognitive-behavioral therapy (CBT) is a psychological method that teaches people how to recognize and change problematic thinking patterns. For women who are suffering emotional difficulties as a result of hormone abnormalities, CBT may be an effective therapy for improving mental health.

CHAPTER THREE

Physical Fitness And Menopausal Health:

Regular physical exercise is a critical component of menopausal wellness. Exercise not only improves general health, but it also helps to manage hormonal changes and accompanying symptoms.

Aerobic activity, such as brisk walking, running, or cycling, has been demonstrated to improve mood and reduce symptoms such as hot flashes. Additionally, aerobic activity improves cardiovascular health, which is especially crucial during menopause.

Strength training is critical for preserving muscle mass and bone density, both of which decrease with age and hormonal changes. Resistance workouts, whether with weights or body weight, may help improve general physical health and well-being.

Yoga, in addition to its significance in mind-body activities, provides mild yet effective physical exertion. It may improve flexibility, balance, and muscular tone while also delivering a sensation of calm and stress reduction.

Individual tastes and fitness levels must be taken into account when designing an exercise plan. Finding pleasant hobbies, such as dance, swimming, or martial arts, promotes commitment to a regular fitness plan, resulting in long-term health advantages.

Sleep Solutions For Good Rest:

Quality sleep is essential for hormone balance and general health. Sleep difficulties are often associated with hormone shifts, especially during menopause.

Implementing good sleep solutions may greatly improve sleep quality.

Creating a regular sleep routine is critical. Going to bed and getting up at the same time every day helps to regulate the body's internal clock, resulting in improved sleep quality. Creating a relaxing nighttime ritual tells the body that it's time to relax.

Creating a pleasant sleeping environment is equally vital. Keeping the bedroom cold, dark, and quiet creates the best circumstances for sleep. Investing in a good mattress and pillows improves overall sleeping comfort.

Limiting caffeine and alcohol consumption, particularly in the hours coming up to bedtime, may improve sleep quality. These chemicals may disrupt the body's normal sleep-wake cycle, leading to sleep disorders.

Before going to bed, try relaxation methods like deep breathing or mild stretching to help you fall asleep. As previously noted, managing stress via mind-body activities may improve sleep quality.

In conclusion, maintaining hormonal balance requires a comprehensive strategy that includes dietary methods, herbal cures, mind-body practices, physical fitness, and sleep solutions. Individuals, especially women going through menopause, may improve their general health and encourage hormonal balance by incorporating these factors into their everyday lives. Consultation with healthcare specialists is vital for tailoring these tactics to individual requirements and ensuring a safe and successful approach to hormonal health.

Menopause is a normal and unavoidable stage in a woman's life, signaling the end of her reproductive years. While it is a normal change, the associated symptoms may be difficult to manage. Many women seek techniques to get through this phase with grace and minimum pain. Managing menopausal symptoms naturally requires a comprehensive strategy that includes lifestyle changes, a supportive mentality, and the maintenance of good relationships, including sexual health and intimacy.

Creating A Supportive Lifestyle.

Adopting a supportive lifestyle during menopause is critical for successful symptom management. Regular exercise, a balanced diet, and enough hydration all play important roles in fostering general well-being. Physical activities such as yoga, walking, and swimming might help relieve symptoms like hot flashes and mood swings. Additionally, adopting a range of nutrient-dense meals high in vitamins and minerals will help with hormone balance and bone health.

Adequate sleep is another essential component of a healthy lifestyle. Menopausal women often have sleep interruptions, which may contribute to weariness and irritation. Creating a suitable sleep environment, practicing relaxation methods, and creating a regular nighttime routine may all help to improve sleep quality.

Menopause requires mindful stress management. Chronic stress may worsen symptoms like anxiety and anger. Stress-relieving activities such as meditation, deep breathing exercises, and journaling might help you maintain emotional balance.

Empowering Your Mindset

The psychological side of menopause is as important. Recognizing and accepting this stage of life is essential for empowering your thinking. Menopause must be seen as a natural process toward knowledge and self-discovery, rather than as a restriction. Maintaining a cheerful attitude may have a big influence on how women face menopause symptoms.

Education and understanding about menopause may help women make more educated health choices. Understanding the hormonal changes that occur in the body at this period might help to explain the accompanying symptoms. This information enables women to proactively manage their health through lifestyle choices and, if required, to seek natural cures or alternative medications.

Self-care habits such as indulging in hobbies, spending quality time with loved ones, and establishing realistic objectives all help to foster a good mentality. Menopause may be a period of personal development and a renewed emphasis on one's health. Embracing the adjustment with resilience and hope may improve the whole experience.

Menopause And Relationships

Navigating menopause entails not just personal adaptations but also concerns for interpersonal connections. Communicating honestly with friends, family, and partners about the physical and emotional changes that occur during menopause promotes understanding and support.

Partners play an important role in fostering a supportive atmosphere. Acknowledging obstacles and honestly addressing issues may help couples improve their relationship. It's important to understand that menopause affects both partners in a relationship. Patience, empathy, and active listening are essential for sustaining strong partnerships.

Educating partners about menopause helps to remove myths and preconceptions, creating a supportive environment. Encouraging open discussion about shifting needs and wants makes both parties feel heard and appreciated. Seeking expert help, such as couples therapy, might provide you with more skills for navigating this transitional period together.

Sexual Health And Intimacy

Menopause may influence sexual health, including libido, vaginal dryness, and general intimacy. Open contact with your healthcare professional is essential for addressing any physical issues.

Maintaining a healthy lifestyle, which includes regular exercise and a well-balanced diet, also helps with general sexual health.

During this stage, it is critical to experiment with different forms of intimacy and communication with your spouse. Understanding each other's needs, being patient, and bringing intimacy into everyday life will help you sustain a pleasant and meaningful relationship.

Experimenting with new types of sexual expression, emphasizing emotional connection, and utilizing water-based lubricants will help resolve any physical changes that may arise. Seeking expert advice from a healthcare physician or a sex therapist may give tailored solutions for maintaining a healthy and fulfilling sexual life after menopause.

To summarize, naturally treating menopausal symptoms requires a complete strategy that includes developing a supportive lifestyle, strengthening your attitude, nourishing relationships, and addressing sexual health and intimacy. Accepting menopause as a transforming period and making educated decisions might result in a happy and rewarding experience.

Women may handle this change with strength and grace by using comprehensive tactics and receiving help as required, enabling themselves to live healthy and productive lives beyond menopause.

CHAPTER FOUR

Managing Changes In Skin And Hair

Menopause is a transitional period in a woman's life that marks the end of her reproductive years. This shift results in a variety of physiological changes, including changes to the skin and hair. Understanding and properly managing these changes is critical for women to go through this phase with confidence and grace.

As women approach menopause, the reduction in estrogen levels has a substantial impact on the changes in their skin and hair.

Estrogen, a hormone released by the ovaries, helps with skin suppleness, collagen formation, and general hydration. With less estrogen, the skin loses part of its firmness and moisture-retaining characteristics.

Wrinkles and fine lines are one of the most visible effects of these hormonal changes. The skin may seem less supple, and reduced collagen synthesis might cause sagging. To combat these effects, a skincare regimen that prioritizes hydration and collagen support is crucial.

Moisturizing becomes an important aspect of skincare throughout menopause. Using products containing hyaluronic acid, glycerin, and other moisturizing components replenishes the skin's moisture levels, resulting in a more youthful and beautiful complexion. Furthermore, integrating retinoids or peptides into your skincare regimen may help stimulate collagen formation and reduce the appearance of fine wrinkles.

Hair, too, changes throughout menopause. Estrogen regulates hair development, and its deficiency may cause hair thinning and loss. The texture of your hair may alter, becoming drier or more brittle. Women may notice that their hair loses the sheen and thickness it formerly had.

To handle these changes, it is essential to follow a nutritious hair care regimen. Using sulfate-free shampoos and conditioners that increase moisture and strengthen the hair shaft may help to enhance hair health. Regular trims assist in handling split ends and avoid additional harm. Additionally, putting hair-strengthening supplements into the diet, such as those containing biotin and omega-3 fatty acids, may help with general hair health.

Bone Health Throughout Menopause

Menopause affects not just the skin and hair, but also the bone health. Estrogen is essential for maintaining bone density, and its loss during menopause increases the risk of osteoporosis and fractures.

The fall in estrogen levels reduces calcium absorption, which is essential for bone health. As a consequence, women approaching menopause must concentrate on maintaining healthy bone density via nutrition, exercise, and, if required, supplements.

Including calcium-rich items in the diet, such as dairy products, leafy green vegetables, and fortified meals, is critical for bone health. Furthermore, vitamin D is required for calcium absorption, and exposure to sunshine or vitamin D supplementation may help keep levels sufficient.

Weight-bearing workouts like walking, running, and strength training are essential for maintaining bone density. These exercises promote bone development and assist in reversing the bone loss associated with menopause. Regular physical exercise promotes bone health while also improving general well-being.

In certain circumstances, doctors may offer bone density tests and, if required, drugs to prevent or cure osteoporosis. Women should have open and proactive talks with their healthcare specialists regarding bone health throughout menopause, as well as explore tailored solutions for keeping strong and healthy bones.

CHAPTER FIVE

Heart Health And Menopause

Menopause-related changes affect not just skin, hair, and bone health, but also cardiovascular health. Estrogen protects the blood arteries and regulates cholesterol levels. Women's cardiovascular health may alter throughout menopause, necessitating attention, and aggressive care due to the decrease in estrogen levels.

Menopause is linked to an increase in cardiovascular risk factors, such as greater LDL cholesterol (also known as "bad" cholesterol), lower HDL cholesterol ("good" cholesterol), and changes in blood vessel function. These variables raise the risk of heart disease and stroke.

Managing heart health during menopause entails making lifestyle modifications that improve cardiovascular health. It is critical to maintain a heart-healthy diet rich in fruits, vegetables, whole grains, and lean proteins yet low in saturated fats. Regular exercise, including aerobic and weight training, improves cardiovascular fitness.

Additionally, stress management is critical for heart health throughout menopause. The hormonal swings and emotional shifts that accompany this period might lead to increased stress, which influences the cardiovascular system.

Regular check-ups with healthcare experts are required to monitor cardiovascular health. Blood pressure, cholesterol levels, and other important indicators should be periodically checked, allowing for early identification and action if required. Women should actively discuss their cardiovascular health with their healthcare providers throughout menopause, as well as seek tailored ways to keep a healthy heart.

Empowering Yourself: Self-Care Practices

As women go through the many changes that occur with menopause, self-care becomes more important. This stage of life allows women to emphasize their physical, emotional, and mental well-being, instilling a feeling of strength and resilience.

Self-care during menopause is a comprehensive strategy that

covers many elements of health. Physical self-care is adopting healthy living habits such as eating a well-balanced diet, exercising regularly, and getting enough sleep. Adequate sleep is especially important during menopause, since hormonal variations may sometimes cause sleep difficulties.

Emotional and mental health are both vital aspects of self-care. Menopause may cause mood swings, anxiety, and other emotional disturbances. Seeking assistance from friends, family, or mental health experts may give important avenues for expression and coping.

Exploring mindfulness and relaxation practices, such as meditation or guided imagery, may help to restore emotional equilibrium. Journaling and self-reflection may be effective techniques for processing ideas and feelings during this transitional phase.

Empowerment through self-care includes accepting the changes that occur with menopause. Celebrating the expertise and experience acquired over time promotes a good perspective. Engaging in activities that offer pleasure and satisfaction, such as following a hobby, spending time in nature, or interacting with loved ones, helps to promote a feeling of purpose and well-being.

Conclusion

Menopause is a normal and unavoidable stage of a woman's life, accompanied by a variety of physical and mental changes. Navigating these changes requires a proactive and comprehensive approach to health and wellness.

Understanding and managing skin and hair changes necessitates personalized skin care and hair care regimens. Accepting these changes as part of the normal aging process might help you feel better about yourself and more confident.

Maintaining bone health throughout menopause requires a mix of nutrition, activity, and, if required, medicinal assistance. Taking preventive measures to maintain bone density promotes long-term skeletal strength and lowers the chance of osteoporosis.

Heart health during menopause is closely related to lifestyle choices such as a heart-healthy diet, regular exercise, stress management, and frequent check-ups with healthcare professionals. These actions jointly improve cardiovascular health and lower the risk of heart disease.

Empowering oneself via self-care activities is an important part of overcoming menopause. Physical, emotional, and mental well-being are all linked, and emphasizing self-care promotes resilience and a good attitude throughout this big life shift.

In essence, menopause is more than simply the end of the reproductive years; it is a chance for women to accept their changing identities with grace and confidence. Understanding the changes, taking preventive steps, and prioritizing self-care may help women traverse menopause with confidence and enter the next chapter of their lives with resilience and energy.